FLAGYL

The Ultimate Guide To Understanding The Use Of Flagy; Exploring The Various Types Of Bacterial And Parasitic Infections, It's Dosage Information And Treatment Duration

Dr. Brent Kai

FLAGYL

Flagyl, also known as metronidazole, is an antibiotic medication used to treat a variety of bacterial infections in the body. It is a powerful drug that works by killing or stopping the growth of bacteria, thereby treating the underlying infection. Flagyl was first discovered in the 1950s by a team of scientists at the pharmaceutical company Rhone-Poulenc in France. Its initial purpose was to treat parasitic infections, but it was eventually found to also be effective against certain types of bacteria. Since then, Flagyl has become a widely used medication and is available in both oral and intravenous forms. Flagyl is a versatile medication and is used to treat infections in different parts of the body, including the stomach, intestines, vagina, and respiratory and skin infections. It is primarily used to treat infections caused by bacteria such as Bacteroides, Clostridium, Fusobacterium, and Peptostreptococcus, among others. One of the most common uses of Flagyl is to treat bacterial vaginosis, a common vaginal infection caused by an overgrowth of harmful bacteria. This condition presents with symptoms such as vaginal discharge, itching, and a bad odor. Flagyl works by restoring the balance of bacteria in the vagina and relieving the symptoms of the infection. Another common use of Flagyl is in the treatment of Helicobacter pylori (H. pylori) infection. H. pylori is a type of bacteria that can cause stomach ulcers and gastritis. Flagyl is often prescribed in combination with other antibiotics to eradicate the bacteria and prevent the recurrence of these conditions. Flagyl is also used to treat infections of the respiratory tract, such as pneumonia, and infections of the skin, bones, and joints. It is also sometimes used to prevent post-surgery infections in some cases. Flagyl is a potent medication, and it works by disrupting the DNA of bacteria, making it impossible for them to grow and cause infection. This makes it an effective treatment for a wide range of bacterial infections. Flagyl is available in both oral and intravenous forms. The oral form is available in tablet, capsule, and liquid formulations, while the intravenous form is administered directly into a vein. The dosage and duration of treatment with Flagyl depend on the type and severity of the infection being treated. When taking Flagyl, it is essential to follow the prescribed dosage and complete the entire course of treatment, even if symptoms improve. Stopping the medication too soon may result in the recurrence of the infection or the development of antibiotic-resistant bacteria. It is also important to take Flagyl with food to reduce the risk of possible stomach upset. Flagyl is generally safe and well-tolerated, like any medication, it may cause some side effects. Common side effects of Flagyl include nausea, stomach upset, diarrhea, headache, and dizziness. These side effects are usually mild and resolve on their own, but if they persist or become severe, it is important to consult a doctor. Flagyl may cause serious side effects such as allergic reactions, blood disorders, and nerve damage. It is important to seek immediate medical attention if any unusual or severe symptoms occur while taking Flagyl. Flagyl should not be used by individuals with a history of hypersensitivity or allergies to metronidazole or other nitroimidazoles. It may also interact with some medications, including blood thinners, anticonvulsants, and alcohol.

Therefore, it is essential to inform your doctor about all the medications you are currently taking before starting treatment with Flagyl. Pregnant and breastfeeding women should also use Flagyl with caution and only under the supervision of a doctor, as it may have potential risks for the fetus or the nursing infant. Studies have shown that Flagyl can pass into breast milk, and it is not recommended for use in infants and young children.

HOW IT WORKS

Flagyl belongs to the class of medications known as

nitroimidazoles, which have potent antimicrobial properties. Its main mode of action is to inhibit the growth and reproduction of the microorganisms causing the infection. The active ingredient in Flagyl, metronidazole, exerts its effects by interfering with the DNA and RNA synthesis of the targeted organisms, which eventually leads to their death. The exact mechanism of action of Flagyl is not fully understood, but it is believed that the medication enters the bacterial or parasitic cells and attaches itself to their DNA. This binding process interferes with the protein synthesis necessary for their survival, thus causing their death. In simpler terms, Flagyl acts as a "molecular hand grenade" that destroys the target organism from the inside out. Flagyl is effective against a wide range of bacteria, including those responsible for common infections such as urinary tract infections, respiratory tract infections, and skin infections. It is also used to treat parasitic and protozoan infections such as trichomoniasis, amoebiasis, and giardiasis. These infections can cause a variety of symptoms, including diarrhea, abdominal pain, and inflammation, which can severely affect a person's daily life if left untreated. Flagyl works by attacking the root cause of these infections, alleviating symptoms, and promoting the healing process. One of the unique qualities of Flagyl is its ability to target a wide range of bacteria and parasites without affecting the beneficial bacteria in the body. This is important because our body's normal flora plays a crucial role in maintaining our overall health. Disrupting this balance can lead to other health issues, such as yeast infections. However, Flagyl does not harm the good bacteria in the body, allowing it to fight off infections effectively without any additional complications. Flagyl is available in various forms, including tablets, capsules, and intravenous (IV) solution. Doctors prescribe the most appropriate form based on the type and severity of the infection, as well as the patient's age and underlying health conditions. Regardless of the form, Flagyl works by entering the bloodstream and circulating throughout the body to reach the site of infection. It is then absorbed by the target microorganisms, leading to their destruction and subsequent elimination from the body. Another critical aspect of how Flagyl works is its ability to penetrate deeply into tissues and body fluids. This is particularly important in treating infections such as bacterial vaginosis, where the microorganisms reside in the vagina's lining and mucus. Flagyl's ability to penetrate and target these hard-to-reach areas makes it a highly effective treatment option for such infections. Flagyl also has anti-inflammatory properties that help reduce swelling and pain caused by these infections. Chronic infections, such as

Crohn's disease and ulcerative colitis, can lead to inflammation and ulceration in the intestinal lining, which can cause severe discomfort and pain. Flagyl helps to reduce this inflammation by targeting the underlying infection, providing relief to the patient. Unlike other antibiotics, Flagyl does not require any activation by enzymes in the body to be effective. This means that it can start working immediately after entering the bloodstream, making it a fast-acting medication. In most cases, patients report feeling relief within a few days of starting treatment with Flagyl. However, to ensure complete eradication of the infection, it is important to complete the full course of treatment as directed by the doctor. Flagyl has been found to be effective in treating infections that are resistant to other antibiotics. This is because it has a unique mechanism of action that is different from traditional antibiotics, making it an effective alternative treatment option. In some cases, Flagyl may be prescribed in combination with other antibiotics to improve its effectiveness against certain microorganisms. Despite its many benefits, Flagyl, like any other medication, can have some side effects. The most common side effects include nausea, vomiting, and loss of appetite. These symptoms are mostly mild and often resolve on their own after a few days of starting treatment. Rare but more severe side effects may include allergic reactions, nerve damage, and liver problems. It is essential to inform the doctor of any adverse reactions experienced while taking Flagyl.

INDICATIONS FOR USE

Flagyl, also known as metronidazole, is a highly effective antibiotic used to treat a wide range of bacterial infections. It has been in use since the 1960s and is recommended by the World Health Organization (WHO) as an essential antibiotic for basic healthcare. Flagyl works by killing or stopping the growth of bacteria and is particularly effective against anaerobic bacteria, which can survive without oxygen. In this article, we will discuss the indications for the use of Flagyl.

Infections caused by bacteria

Flagyl is commonly used to treat various infections caused by bacteria. These include infections of the skin, stomach, intestines, joints, and respiratory tract. It is effective against both gram-positive and gram-negative bacteria, making it a versatile treatment option for a wide range of bacterial infections. Some of the common bacterial infections that can be treated with Flagyl include bacterial vaginosis, pelvic inflammatory disease, and bacterial pneumonia.

Protozoal infections

Aside from bacteria, Flagyl is also effective against protozoal infections, which are caused by tiny organisms such as amoeba and giardia. These infections can affect different parts of the body, including the digestive tract, genitals, and respiratory system. Flagyl works by weakening the protozoa's cell walls, which eventually leads to their death. It is often used to treat infections such as amoebiasis, trichomoniasis, and giardiasis.

Dental and oral infections

Flagyl can be prescribed to treat dental and oral infections caused by bacteria. These include dental abscesses, gingivitis, and periodontitis. Dental abscesses occur when bacteria infect the inner part of the tooth, leading to inflammation and pus accumulation. Flagyl can effectively kill the bacteria causing the abscess and aid in the healing process. Gingivitis and periodontitis are gum infections that can also be treated with Flagyl.

Post-surgical infections

Infections can occur after a surgical procedure, especially if proper sterilization measures were not taken. Flagyl is often prescribed before and after surgery to prevent and treat possible infections. It is commonly used in surgical procedures involving the digestive tract, genitals, and reproductive system. The bacteria present in these areas can cause life-threatening infections if not treated promptly.

Bacterial septicemia

Bacterial septicemia is a severe infection of the bloodstream caused by bacteria. It can occur due to untreated or severe infections in other parts of the body, such as pneumonia, meningitis, or urinary tract infections. Flagyl is used as part of the treatment for bacterial septicemia, along with other antibiotics and supportive care. It helps to eliminate the bacteria from the bloodstream and prevent further spread of the infection.

Antibiotic-associated diarrhea

Antibiotic use can sometimes kill the beneficial bacteria in the gut, allowing harmful bacteria such as Clostridium difficile (C. diff) to thrive. This can lead to diarrhea and inflammation of the large intestine, known as antibiotic-associated diarrhea. Flagyl is often prescribed to treat this condition, as it is particularly effective against C. diff. It works by inhibiting the growth and reproduction of C. diff, allowing

the gut's natural bacteria to regain
balance.

H. pylori infection

H. pylori is a type of bacteria that
can cause chronic gastritis, a
condition that involves
inflammation of the stomach
lining. This infection can also lead
to stomach ulcers and is a
significant risk factor for stomach
cancer. Flagyl is used in
combination with other antibiotics
to treat H. pylori infection and
heal stomach ulcers. It is typically
prescribed for a few weeks, along
with acid-reducing medications to
promote healing.

Crohn's disease

Flagyl is sometimes used as a treatment for Crohn's disease, a chronic inflammatory bowel disease that affects the digestive tract. It is believed that the anti-inflammatory properties of Flagyl may help reduce inflammation in the gut, improving symptoms such as abdominal pain, diarrhea, and rectal bleeding. However, the use of Flagyl for Crohn's disease is still under investigation and may not be effective in all cases.

Bacterial vaginosis and other vaginal infections

Vaginal infections such as bacterial vaginosis and trichomoniasis are commonly caused by an imbalance of bacteria in the vagina. Flagyl can effectively treat these infections by killing the harmful bacteria and allowing the normal, healthy bacteria to thrive. It may be prescribed as a vaginal gel or cream for local treatment or taken orally for more severe infections.

Parasitic skin infections

Flagyl can also be used to treat skin infections caused by parasites such as Giardia or Demodex. These infections can cause itching, redness, and inflammation of the skin. Flagyl helps to eliminate the parasites, providing relief from the symptoms. It is also used to treat rosacea, a chronic skin condition characterized by redness and inflammation on the face.

DOSAGE AND ADMINISTRATION

Dosage and administration refer to the process of correctly prescribing and administering medication to patients. It is a crucial aspect of healthcare as the correct dosage and route of administration can ensure optimal therapeutic benefits and prevent adverse effects. Dosage refers to the amount of medication prescribed to a patient, while administration is the method by which the medication is delivered into the body. The dosage and administration of medication are determined by various factors, including the patient's age, weight, medical condition, and the medication's pharmacological properties. The first step in prescribing medication is determining the correct dosage. This is done by considering the therapeutic range of the medication, which is the range of doses that have been proven to be effective and safe for the majority of patients. The dosage can vary depending on the patient's condition, as well as other factors such as drug interactions and any underlying medical conditions. In most cases, the dosage is determined by the weight of the patient. Children and adults have different doses of medication due to their varying body weights and developmental stages. For example, a child's dose of a medication may be calculated using their body weight, while an adult's dose may be a fixed amount based on the medication's pharmacokinetic properties.

Dosage can also be affected by factors such as renal or hepatic impairment, as these conditions may affect the body's ability to metabolize and excrete the medication. Another important consideration in dosage is the frequency of administration. This refers to how often a patient should take their medication, and it can vary from once a day to multiple times a day, depending on the medication's duration of action. Some medications have a longer duration of action and can be taken less frequently, while others need to be taken more often to maintain therapeutic levels.

There are different routes of administration for medication, which include oral, topical, inhalation, subcutaneous, intramuscular, and intravenous routes. Each route has its advantages and disadvantages, and the choice of route depends on factors such as the patient's medical condition, the urgency of treatment, and the medication's pharmacokinetic properties. One of the most common routes of administration is the oral route, which involves swallowing medication in liquid or tablet form. It is a convenient route of administration and is suitable for patients who can swallow and digest medication. The absorption of medication through the oral route can be affected by factors such as the medication's stability in the acidic environment of the stomach and any food or drinks consumed together with the medication. The topical route involves the application of medication onto the skin or mucous membranes, such as the nose, eyes, and vagina. This route is commonly used for medications such as creams, ointments, and eye drops. The absorption of medication through the topical route is usually slower compared to other routes, but it can be effective for localized conditions. Inhalation is another route of administration that involves the delivery of medications directly to the lungs. This route is suitable for patients with respiratory conditions such as asthma and chronic obstructive pulmonary disease (COPD). Medications administered through inhalation act quickly and can be effective in managing acute symptoms. The subcutaneous and intramuscular routes involve the administration of medications into the fatty tissue beneath the skin and the muscle, respectively. These routes are commonly used for medications that need to be slowly released into the body, such as insulin and vaccines. The absorption of medication through these routes can be affected by factors such as the location and depth of the injection, as well as the patient's muscle mass. Intravenous administration involves the direct delivery of medication into the vein. This route is used in emergency situations or when immediate effects of the medication are needed. Intravenous administration is also used for medications that cannot be taken orally or those that have a narrow therapeutic index, meaning that the difference between a therapeutic dose and a toxic dose is small. Once the correct dosage and route of administration have been determined, it is essential to educate the patient on how to take their medication properly. This includes providing information on the dosage, frequency of administration, possible side effects, and any food or drink interactions that need to be avoided. Patient education is crucial in ensuring medication compliance and promoting positive therapeutic outcomes.

WARNINGS AND PRECAUTIONS

Warnings:

Allergic reactions:

One of the most important warnings associated with Flagyl is the risk of allergic reactions. Some individuals may be allergic to metronidazole or other ingredients in the medication. Allergic reactions to Flagyl can range from mild to severe, and may include symptoms such as skin rash, hives, itching, swelling, difficulty breathing, and anaphylactic shock. It is important to inform your doctor if you have any history of allergies before starting Flagyl.

Neurological effects:

Flagyl has been known to cause neurological side effects in some patients. These may include dizziness, vertigo, headaches, and coordination problems. In some rare cases, Flagyl may also cause more serious neurological effects such as seizures, confusion, hallucinations, and nerve damage. It is important to monitor for any changes in neurological status and to seek medical attention if any concerning symptoms arise.

Blood disorders:

Flagyl may also have an effect on the blood cells, leading to potential disorders such as leukopenia (low white blood cell count), neutropenia (low neutrophil count), and thrombocytopenia (low platelet count). These blood disorders can increase the risk of infection, bleeding, and other complications. Therefore, individuals with a history of blood disorders should inform their doctor before starting treatment with Flagyl.

Alcohol interaction:

It is important to avoid consumption of alcohol while

taking Flagyl. Mixing alcohol and Flagyl can lead to unpleasant side effects such as nausea, vomiting, abdominal cramps, flushing, and headache. It is recommended to avoid alcohol for at least 48 hours after the last dose of Flagyl to prevent these adverse reactions.

Drug interactions:

Flagyl can interact with several medications, leading to potentially serious complications. Some medications that may interact with Flagyl include blood thinners, anticonvulsants, lithium, and certain HIV medications. It is important to disclose all medications, including over-the-counter drugs and supplements, to your doctor before starting Flagyl to prevent these interactions.

Precautions:

Pregnancy and breastfeeding:

Flagyl is classified as a pregnancy category B medication, which means it is generally considered safe to use during pregnancy. However, it is always important to inform your doctor if you are pregnant or planning to become pregnant before starting any medication. Flagyl can also pass into breast milk, so it is recommended to consult with a doctor before taking this medication while breastfeeding.

Liver and kidney disease:

Individuals with a history of liver disease or kidney disease may require a dose adjustment or closer monitoring while taking Flagyl. This is because the medication is primarily metabolized in the liver and excreted by the kidneys. Any impairment in these organs can affect the way Flagyl is processed and may increase the risk of adverse reactions.

Central nervous system (CNS) disorders:

Flagyl may worsen certain CNS disorders such as epilepsy and multiple sclerosis. It is important to inform your doctor if you have a history of these disorders before starting treatment with Flagyl.

Peripheral neuropathy:

Flagyl has been associated with cases of peripheral neuropathy, a nerve disorder that can cause tingling, numbness, and weakness in the limbs. If you experience any symptoms of peripheral neuropathy while taking Flagyl, it is important to inform your doctor immediately.

Use in children:

Flagyl is usually not recommended for use in children under the age of 18, unless specifically prescribed by a doctor. This is because there is limited research on the safety and efficacy of Flagyl in pediatric patients.